Walberg

678 357
3443

Enough Drugs! I Am a Woman and Can Heal Naturally

Gedalou

Enough Drugs! I Am a Woman and Can Heal Naturally

a practical guide to feeling your best

Gedalia Genin PhD

ISBN: 0692811613
ISBN 13: 9780692811610

Acknowledgements

To my grandmother, Bertha Tarlow, for her strength, courage and strong hands and whose love was crucial in my early years.

To my husband, David, whose unconditional love and friendship is like a rock of stability for me.

To our children, Zachary and Noah, who gave me the greatest gift of my life—motherhood! Your presence awakened my desire for a holistic lifestyle, "a beautiful life" as my son put it.

To the Siddha Yoga Path for the practices and teachings that give me the strength to move forward each day with joy and creativity.

To Vasant Lad who I am blessed to have as my Ayurvedic teacher and for his unconditional love and healing energy.

To Dr. Michael Mamas for all I learned as a healer.

To Dr. Taz who believed and trusted in me to share my gifts with her patients.

To nature which is radiant, beautiful, alive and life sustaining!

To the power of colors that transform my vision every day.

To Gali Kronenberg — a wiz with words, and a talent for drawing out my best ideas. Gali has been an amazing editor, mentor, and guide. You ushered me back to my own voice. Your clarity and insight helped me distill the gems I've learned over a lifetime about healing and wellness.

"Each day of our lives we need to find the strength that allows us to take action with fierce love. We need the strength to dust off the mirror of our consciousness and show up in ways that go beyond what we feel like or don't feel like to fulfill our greater purpose and destiny.

For this, we need a guide, a mentor, a healer, a compassionate listener, a safe environment; an attunement to our very own nature.

This is who I am and this is how I can serve you."

—Gedalia

Disclaimer: The information in this book is designed to provide helpful information on the subjects discussed. This book is not meant to be used, nor should it be used, to diagnose or treat any medical condition. For diagnosis or treatment of any medical problem, consult your own physician. The publisher and author are not responsible for any specific health or allergy needs that may require medical supervision and are not liable for any damages or negative consequences from any treatment, action, application or preparation, to any person reading or following the information in this book. References are provided for informational purposes only and do not constitute an endorsement of any websites or other sources. Readers should be aware that the websites listed in this book may change. The names in the stories have been changed.

Introduction

We live in an age of casual pill popping. The Journal of the American Medical Association warns of "significant increases in overall prescription drug use" that is unrelated to our aging population. This frenzy of prescription-drug taking is abetted by doctors, patients and, of course, Big Pharma – eager to protect a U.S. drug market worth more than $350 billion a year.

Whatever ails us – a desire to lose weight, alleviate depression or ease anxiety – Americans reach for a pill. It's not just men or women over 50 relying on meds. Teens are dosing up early and often – and not just on marijuana. Come midterms or finals, prices for individual pills of Vicodin, OxyContin and Ritalin spike.

This guide isn't about demonizing prescription drugs. It is about learning daily holistic approaches that lend toward "healing," not fixing a broken part. Everything in this guide empowers women with healthy effective alternatives.

Often our symptoms are our body's way of speaking to us and are a wakeup call to change our behavior, approach or attitude. When we take medications that mask our symptoms and dull our emotions we dim our ability to recognize the underlying problem and what our body or heart is trying to tell us. Our body and emotions impart critical feedback. Sometimes, it's an urgent call to make a much–needed change.

Emotional pain can cut deep and hurt and can push us to grow and heal. Yes, there are times when medication – be it an antidepressant or antibiotic– is the right course. Antibiotics are crucial for bacterial infections and in no way, am I telling you to stop using them or even anti-depressants. But at best, these are temporary solutions. Healing involves new healthful behaviors and practices. A Band-Aid approach of pills does not heal the root cause of symptoms nor does it address the whole person.

The two powerful figures in my life – my mother, and my grand-mother– embodied opposite qualities, one shadow, and the other light. While it was my grandmother who I always loved, enjoyed and admired, it was my mother's emotional and physical suffering, and it's weight on the rest of the family, that sent me on a path to my calling to work as a holistic healer and artist.

My mother not only couldn't cook; she didn't know how to nourish. Instead of appreciating her own mother's warmth towards her children, she resented it. My mom suffered from debilitating rheumatoid arthritis. Her daily medications were lined up like soldiers along the kitchen counter. The meds kept her going but never addressed the frustration, resentment, and anger she felt for having been denied the real career she'd wanted. In her perspective, she was "trapped at home in the suburbs with four small kids" while she yearned for a more glamorous life.

My father was adamant that she remain a homemaker. When she died from a brain tumor after taking powerful arthritis meds for more than forty years, he blamed the drug companies and was bent on suing them. We talked him out of it.

Despite the pain in our relationship, it was from my long-suffering mother that I learned the lesson that health is a choice and that to heal is a choice. I can see now that she acted on the information and understanding that was available to her at the time. I don't know that if she had stopped her hefty daily dosage of rheumatoid arthritis medications, her illness would have been cured. There was simply no recognition at the time that addressing the emotional aspects of her illness might have soothed her physical health and mental anguish.

By contrast, my grandmother's world was filled with love, joy and an appreciation of life's rituals. The aroma of cooked fruit on my grandmother's stove remains a strong memory. We visited her Brooklyn apartment every Sunday and returned to North Woodmere, on Long Island New York, with half a dozen mason jars of peaches, strawberries or whatever fruit she had canned that week.

Bertha would climb atop a stepping stool to reach the upper shelves of her cupboards where they were stored, calling down to us to "take more." Though not a wealthy woman, in her world, there was always "enough" and plenty to share with friends, neighbors, and family.

Even as a girl, I admired her courage and strength coming to this country by herself speaking no English, fleeing Eastern Europe when the hope of life was slim during World War II. As a teen, she fileted fish with her bare hands at the Fulton Street Fish Market in the Bowery in New York City, after arriving by boat from Russia.

Something else I marveled at watching my grandmother – beyond her generosity and work ethic – was the pleasure she took in her daily rituals. Every morning after her prayers, she walked from her apartment to the butcher and grocer to shop for fresh food. She didn't go out of her way to exercise, but she never learned to drive, and loved any chance to be out in the fresh air.

She didn't perceive the hours she spent preparing bone broths, roasting vegetables, whole chickens, and briskets every week as a labor, but as acts of love to nourish her family. This isn't to imply that women belong in the kitchen. But what my grandmother's life taught me was the importance of taking pleasure in the rhythms and rituals of our daily lives. With the right understanding, rituals help us to stay grounded and nourish our bodies, minds, and hearts.

When I think back to the birth of my first son Zack, I realize that I unconsciously modeled my life on my grandmother's. My husband and I had made the decision to move from Brewster, a Westchester County suburb, to a small town in upstate New York called Hudson. We found an old home with high ceilings, original tall windows, and 19th-century pegboard floors. We were fortunate to purchase a "fire sale" from a bank foreclosure on an 1860's row house, a block from the Hudson River. Disheveled as it was from the outside, we could see its potential.

Looking back, the choice to shift the pace of our lives from the whirlwind of stress and financial pressures we'd felt in the city was the first step on my own path to healing.

My husband and I embraced the labor of refinishing the old wide board floors and long wood staircase (like my grandmothers) and hired painters and an architect to help us restore the property to its original Victorian beauty. Each room was painted a vibrant color reflecting that period.

For the first time in my adult life, we had an edible garden in our backyard and our kids could walk to a nearby park to watch the boats sail past on the river. The community wasn't gentrified and I loved the mix of people around us as well as the many artists flocking up from Manhattan on the weekends. That year, 1988, was the same time we discovered a meditation and yoga retreat an hour and a half away that became a regular part of our lives. We visited most weekends and began to discover a life-changing depth of inner quiet and serenity. Though my grandmother lived in New York City, it felt as if the choices I was making in my life were inspired by hers.

I feel deep within my heart and in my being, that it was Bertha's love that helped shape who I am today.

While the lifestyle choice to live in a small town in view of the Hudson River and Catskill mountains was a great boon, it was the journey that unfolded through meditation that showed me that inner peace and well-being exist within each of us. My discovery of my passion to serve as a healer unfolded through meditation. And it was the birth of our children that gave birth to my passion for a holistic lifestyle.

Creativity

"Here's a startling fact," writes Dr. Jay Kumar in his book, *Brain, Body & Being*. "In our modern, 24/7 high-tech world, the average person is bombarded with the equivalent of 174 newspapers of data every day! That's five times the amount of sensory information a person received just 30 years ago."

No wonder we feel exhausted, overwhelmed and stressed. The busy habit is a warped status symbol, a humble brag of CEOs, stay-at-home moms and dads and of anyone convinced their workplace or home would collapse without them.

This busyness addiction isn't simply a function of the workplace. Once we return home, Kumar writes, "We can't quit our e-habit. Even in our bedrooms, living rooms, even bathrooms, we peruse our screens, feeling the need to check email, Facebook, Twitter or Instagram."

In my own life, I've discovered that one drug-free, simple, and playful way to heal the emotional and physical toll of this cacophony of distraction is one many of us last pursued in childhood — coloring, painting, and dancing!

In short — the antidote is creativity. Creative expression heals! No matter if you feel inspired to play the piano, pen a poem, paint with watercolors or whirl like a dervish. This isn't New Age woo-woo. It's the analysis of more than 100 research studies reviewed by the American Journal of Public Health in the study, *The Connection Between Art, Healing, and Public Health*.

In "Make More Art: The Health Benefits of Creativity," James Clear writes in the Huffington Post, "Creating art doesn't just make you feel better, it also creates real, physical changes inside your body." His account of our predicament mirrors numerous other studies cited by Dr. Kumar.

"In our always-on, always-connected world of television, social media, and on-demand everything, it can be stupidly easy to spend your entire day consuming information and simply responding to all the inputs that bombard your life," writes Clear.

"Art offers an outlet and a release from all of that. Take a minute to ignore all the incoming signals and create an outgoing one instead. Produce something. Express yourself in some way. If you contribute rather than consume, anything you do can be a work of art.

"Open a blank document and start typing. Put pen to paper and sketch a drawing. Grab your camera and take a picture. Turn up the music and dance. Start a conversation and make it a good one.

"Build something. Share something. Craft something. Cut out pictures for a collage. Make more art. Your health and happiness will improve and we'll all be better off for it."

In summary, Clear concludes, these studies demonstrate that creative pursuits "redirect our focus, and distract us from thoughts of grief, stress or physical pain."

Creative expression not only benefits our mood but our physical body as well. A 2004 study published in the *Journal of Psychosomatic Medicine* demonstrated how creative writing has been shown to boost the immune system for people with HIV. In other words, creative expression doesn't just make you feel better, it also creates real, physical changes inside your body.

My own experience is that connecting with my inner artist through meditation was akin to finding my own personal Eden.

When I paint, I experience it as a kind of bath for my mind. Much like meditation, being with color, shifts my relationship with time. When I tap my unbridled imagination, I find I drop into an experience of flow. I've found that it's when I'm alone with my paints and brushes that I truly experience God's presence within.

The blank canvas is a metaphor for the daily opportunity to invent our life and fill it in anew.

Even daydreaming has been discovered by neuroscience to enhance creativity and productivity. The mere act of allowing your mind to wander opens a space for creative ideas. The next time you are washing dishes or making your bed notice what comes up. Steven Spielberg wrote he received his greatest movie ideas while driving.

What if I don't feel like I'm a creative person?

Expand your concept of creativity. Creativity embraces far more than painting. You can be creative in the way you cook, dance or decorate your home. Your creative niche may be a craft: knitting, making jewelry, woodworking or scrapbooking.

Life offers us untold opportunities to express our creativity. While I love to set aside time to paint, I look for moments throughout my day to feel creative. It may be the way I choose to dress, the flowers I arrange in a vase or my original twist on a favorite recipe. Or it may be cutting out a picture from a magazine or a phrase that inspires me. Yes, it's OK to play!

Tech too often turns us into Zombie-like consumers of culture. But if used consciously, our cell phones or iPads can also be a vehicle for creative play. You may wish to use your phone as a vessel to see and notice the beauty that surrounds you. The same street you walk along every day may look new if you're attuned to the play of light and shadow. Each of us sees the world differently, and photography is one means to share with others our distinct way of seeing and experiencing the world around us.

All of us, professional and amateur, share an impulse to create. Break free from the straightjacket of creating art only if it makes money. There's validity to art, even if we never exhibit our work or win awards. Creativity is an essential part of what it is to be alive.

Painting – not pills – relieved my own chronic back pain and grief. I literally felt that painting, and in my case, painting with lots of bright, vivid colors, released tension and lifted my spirits. Today, more and more, psychologists and therapists prescribe various forms of artistic expression to patients. For you, it may not be painting. Some of my client's report feeling greater enthusiasm for life from penning the story of their lives, creating a performance piece or through dance. Creativity can be a kind of alchemy for our emotions.

It is healing to have an emotional remove from actual events. Telling our stories is how we see connections and gain perspective on our past and it can serve as a lens onto the present.

Many of my clients tell me that keeping a journal or making family album photos is a form of therapy. Creativity is also a healthy and safe way to release grief or shame.

If you're daunted by oil paints, watercolor or writing, pick up a crayon or marker. In 2016, Dr. Nikki Martinez wrote in the Huffington Post that coloring books for adults are great for mental and emotional health. Coloring, she writes, "ring us back to a simpler time. An activity that invokes carefree and happier memories of childhood."

There's nothing "New Age" about creativity. Renowned Swiss psychologist Carl Jung gave his adult patients a "prescription" to paint and draw. Jung thought it would help his patient's "access their subconscious and new self-knowledge," writes Martinez.

Let creativity serve as a pathway to discover what inspires and brings you joy. Jung also encouraged his patients to paint *mandalas*, a

Sanskrit word meaning center, circumference or sacred circle. Jung believed that mandalas denote a unification of opposites, serve as expressions of the Self, and represent the sum of who we are. Painting mandalas were central to Jung's own therapeutic practice. He said he found creating them served as a "path to the center."

A child's circle may be her earliest representation of the self. According to the Yogic masters, humankind's greatest goal is to overcome the cosmic illusion that all forms of life are separate and distinct. A mandala depicts the truth in microcosm, beyond the polarities of day and night, life and death, good and evil, pleasure and pain, light and shadow. A mandala writes Judith Cornell, depicts the "totality of God's absolute nature."

"We are born through a circular opening pushed out by a series of circular muscles to a planet which is spinning in a circular orbit around the sun," writes Cornell.

Creative expression can help us access our own inner knowing and intelligence. Think of mandalas as a visual meditation, a diagram of the cosmos.

Mandalas can draw our awareness to a spiritual truth that is hard to grasp with the mind. Even if the mind doesn't know why, you may experience the mandala as soothing and calming, much the same as the rose-tinted stain glass windows of a cathedral may infuse you with a feeling of awe or calm.

During the chaotic years of WWI, Jung wrote: "When I began drawing the Mandalas ... I saw that everything, all the paths I had been following, all the steps I had taken, was leading back to a single point-namely, to the midpoint." He went on to call it "the path to the center."

It's also said that mandalas activate the seven energy centers of the body known as *chakras*, which are depicted as wheels. Deep meditators report having the inner visualization that each chakra is itself its own mandala.

Austrian philosopher, social reformer and architect Rudolph Steiner who developed Waldorf Education, emphasized the importance for children to make things by hand. Waldorf schools are noted for their knitting classes, drawing and learning through movement. When my own son, Zack, attended a Waldorf school in the Berkshires, I recall watching in fascination children learning math at an early age through "clapping hands." It was an example that learning can take place with the whole body, not just the head. Steiner wrote that working with our hands can usher us into a state of flow.

If you don't give a lot of credence to Austrian philosophers, consider the finding that CEOs identified creativity as "the single most important leadership competency for enterprises seeking a path through this complexity" according to a new study by IBM."

Creativity allows us to embrace experimentation and originality. Our culture prizes results. But often it takes play to access genius. Let creativity become your meditation, your warm, soothing bath, if you will, for your mind. It can be as simple as letting a colored pen and a sketchpad distract us from the drumbeat of negative thoughts.

Your soul wants to speak, and often it does so through creative expression.

Donna, a 50-year-old mother of teenagers, came to the practice seeking help in balancing her hormones. Her hot flashes were to the tune of five or more a day. She was referred to me from one of the integrative doctors to support her emotional well-being as she suffered depression, anxiety and overwhelm. After one of our first sessions, I asked her if she had once painted as I sensed her artistic abilities just looking at the way she dressed and overall style. She shared several paintings she had done from photos on her iPhone as if she was pulling out hidden gems from a treasure chest. I was in awe. No wonder she felt depressed. She rarely expressed her artistic passion. Within a few energy healing sessions, having her use essential oils such as clary sage, ylang ylang and sweet orange and an Ayurvedic diet with enough protein, her anxiety, and hot flashes diminished to once per day. At each of our energy sessions, I reminded her to make art—daily. She soon began showing me with great joy what she created. She even began to visualize paintings during our sessions. As art became an integral part of her life, she was better able to follow the dietary and herbal protocols from both the doctors and myself and began to feel more balanced, vibrant and more like herself.

Meditation

How do I approach meditation?

Does meditation scare you? The thought of a "no thought" state may strike you as impossible. The idea of ridding yourself of the thicket of thoughts racing through your head may sound as onerous as weeding an overgrown garden! My clients lament: "My mind is always racing." "I can't turn off my thoughts." "Endless to-do lists loop through my brain."

In actuality, meditation doesn't involve controlling or uprooting thoughts. Quite the contrary, it takes a gentler approach akin to wading in a pool of water or floating on a raft. The simple practice of sitting (lying down works, too) in stillness and just "being" doesn't have to involve effort. Sure, situations and scenarios may continue to play out in your mind as you sit and meditate. But one approach to meditation involves simply watching your thoughts rather than grabbing onto them. You simply witness them.

We all have thoughts, even longtime meditators. The issue isn't whether you have thoughts when you meditate but your ability to witness in stillness and watch them as they rise and fall. There's no need to indulge your mental activity. One of the benefits of meditation is you may no longer feel so intensely identified with the you that is thinking.

This is what's known as witness consciousness. This practice provides benefits off your meditation cushion as well. When a challenge arises, you possess the strength to take it in without flying into high drama. You may need to act, but you can do so with calm, clarity and ease.

I always share with people, and urge my children, not to wait for a crisis to start meditating. I discovered the truth of this in my own life.

One day, my husband and I learned his business partner had laundered our money. He was sent to prison but this still left us to face devastating real-world consequences. We lost our home, cars, and rental properties. In our fifties, we had to start from scratch. We had to trade our beautiful 5,000-square-foot home for a tiny apartment. I had to take a full-time job and work weekends, as did my husband. The temptation to blame, quarrel or wallow in victimhood was enormous! We had our moments.

Faced with this dire situation, I saw no way out but to double-down on my meditation and other spiritual practices. One profound source of comfort was prayer. Fortunately, my husband and I weren't trying to learn to move into stillness and meditate for the first time at the height of this drama. We both had a steady meditation practice. I'd say it saved our marriage.

There was no denying things were stressful. Yet I found meditation, as well as practices like chanting, and my art inoculated me from feeling choked or subsumed by our financial challenges. Indeed, with my mind at peace, and faith in my heart, I began to notice miracles everywhere. What we needed simply began to show up. We felt the generosity of our friends. Even strangers showed us a great deal of kindness. I wasn't used to this—receiving a helping hand. I was accustomed to "living atop the hill" so to speak. I was always the giver. Now, I was the one receiving.

If not for our years of meditation, I think we would have cracked – or at least not stayed together as a couple. While we relied on each other, we found that meditation helped us to find the inner strength to trust and perceive the divine protection that is always present. I began to see our situation as an opportunity to let go of fear. It was as if I was being shown that something terrible could happen, and I'd still be fine.

Our egos still wanted to blame. I know it was the spiritual practices we had built up for so long prior to this event that saved us.

I always created a sacred space in all the places we lived. Even with our more demanding work schedules, my husband and I found time to meditate and pray each day. The inner stillness we experienced began to feel like an enormous treasure. More than ever before, we found an attitude of gratitude began to permeate our consciousness.

Meditation & Surfing

Imagine a surfer riding a wave. Her challenge is to stay aloft as waves crash and churn beneath her and let them carry her to smooth water.

It's an apt metaphor for meditation. Too many people quit before they are carried into the smooth waters of inner stillness. They notice their churning thoughts and hop off before finding balance and stillness. Just like a surfer, you need to ride through those first choppy waters - no matter, if your mind races for the first ten minutes. Ride out those thoughts and you'll find periods of deep calm and stillness. No need to judge the choppy parts. It's all part of the journey to inner peace.

Do I need to change my religion to meditate?

Clients often ask, "Do I need to chant Om to meditate?" No, you don't. You can believe in Jesus, Allah, Buddha or some other deity and still meditate. Meditation isn't a religion, it's a state of consciousness. Clients often tell me when they garden, knit or cook it feels as if they're meditating. It is true that when one does anything with a one-pointed focus it feels like meditation. There are certainly benefits to playing tennis, the flute, cooking or performing any activity with total focus, and there are still unique and powerful benefits to sitting to meditate.

Three Types of Meditation

1. Guided Meditation
This is a perfect place to begin. There are easily thousands of audio recordings, videos, even animations with music or verbal instructions to guide you into meditation.

It's great to experiment and see what type of guided meditation suits you, and you may discover, it varies by the day. One reason there are so many types of meditation is that there are so many disparate types of meditators. Some guided meditations may ask you to visualize a placid lake or a column of light or a placid scene.

2. Empty Bowl Meditation
This style of Ayurvedic meditation is one where you sit with your palms open, resting on your thighs, facing upwards. As you sit, focus on releasing negative thoughts and emotions while watching the "space" between the breath. You may wish to repeat a mantra, a sacred utterance in Sanskrit. One powerful mantra is *Soham*, which means, "I am That." One chants this to shift one's sense of self to identify with the universe or ultimate reality.

Experiment repeating *Soham* on the in breath and then the out breath. The open hands represent the "giving up" of negative thinking and opening to positive energy. Your hands or some other part of your body may feel tingly and that's a good sign indicating subtle energy is awake and flowing.

3. Chakra Meditation

This is a great meditation for visual meditators. I recommend a CD called "Toning the Chakras" by Joy Gardner Gordon. I use this CD in my Holistic Approach to Grief and Loss class. Chakras are vibrational centers of energy in the subtle body. These seven centers, also known as "wheels of energy" or "wheels of light," are located from the base of the spine to the crown of the head in the subtle body. They directly affect the state of our mental, physical and spiritual health.

By clearing the chakras one gains access to more energy, a feeling of lightness and overall improved health.

You may also take the help of sound for meditation. The tambura, a four-stringed lute, is an ancient droning instrument originating in India that has long been used for meditation and yoga to aid in quieting the mind. In the Keys to The Heart Meditation Series, Master Tambura Player Betty McKeon plays this beautiful instrument in seven key resonances referred to as base notes. You can find these CDs on Amazon.

Is meditation a spiritual practice?

"Meditation is not religion, not spirituality—it's a technology of upgrading the mind that can enrich one's life, including one's religious life," writes Jay Michaelson, author of *Evolving Dharma*." We're used to the idea of physical fitness. Time to get used to the idea of contemplative fitness, and practice at least as diligently."

In *Meditation as a Spiritual Practice*, Genevieve Paulson writes: "Meditation has many purposes: healing, past life awareness, mental clarity, and relaxation. This practice can also enhance our spiritual lives by bringing about peak experiences or transcendental states. Meditation as a spiritual practice focuses on expanding consciousness and awareness." The techniques in her book can also help develop clairvoyance, clairaudience, and other psychic abilities.

What are some of the proven benefits of meditation?

In her book, *A Mind of Your Own*, Dr. Kelly Brogan, holistic psychiatrist, lists meditations many proven medical benefits. "Meditation is just as effective as antidepressant drugs in treating anxiety or depression, but without the side effects, according to a study conducted by researchers from Johns Hopkins University that was published in the journal JAMA Internal Medicine." Meditation calms the mind, relieves stress, and can enhance intuition and creativity.

How can I prepare for meditation?

Pranayama or breath work.

The word "prana" means breath. However, according to the yogic texts, this refers to more than just oxygen. Prana is our life force. It is the vital force that bathes every cell in our being.

Yogis have long used different breathing techniques to heal the body, mind and to prepare for meditation. Pranayama is a practice to help control the breath.

You can learn pranayama from a skilled yoga teacher or Ayurvedic practitioner. One great side effect is that it helps tone the belly!

Although yogic breathing can seem daunting to some, I recommend a simple breath practice to my clients. It's called "deep belly breathing."

Simply hold your hand on your belly while sitting up or lying down as you inhale fill the belly like you are filling a balloon. Push the stomach out on the inhale to the count of five. Then exhale to the count of five. The idea is to breathe more deeply from the bottom of the lungs, not only from the top of the chest. This is how babies breathe. This increase of oxygen in the body has many benefits. I like to call it Vitamin "O" as it bathes the cells in vital energy. It's the most renewable energy we have if we pay attention to it.

There are various yogic breath techniques that you can learn on YouTube with Ayurvedic doctor, Dr. Vasant Lad and other teachers. Simply search "pranayama."

Sophie a 35-year-old nurse came to our integrative office because of panic attacks. After many years of anti-anxiety meds, she felt frustrated and anxious. Her breath was short and convulsive at times. Little by little her deep sense of fear began to dissipate after learning how to breathe.

Where is the best place to meditate?

This too is part of the discovery that awaits you as you embark on meditation. You need to find or create your own "best place" to meditate. Typically, this is a quiet place where you won't be disturbed.

The place where you meditate will begin to hold the vibrations and positive energy you have cultivated there so that when you return to sit on your mat or chair you can glide more easily into a place of serenity.

I find it's helpful to create a sacred space in your home or in a backyard studio. If you don't have an extra room, then a closet or corner in your bedroom will suffice. The main thing is that it is your space, your personal sacred sanctuary.

Just like a gardener tills the soil to prepare for planting, in the same way, the regular practice of meditation in your own space fertilizes the ground underneath you so that when you sit you reap the energy you have accumulated there.

A few basic elements you'll want are a chair or cushion, a candle, perhaps a crystal or an image of the Buddha, Christ or the image of a spiritual teacher or master who inspires you. Indeed, you may wish to include a photo of yourself on your altar.

You can find colorful meditation cushions, gemstones or essential oils online. I find the colored gemstones I've put in my meditation room heighten the vibratory energy of the space. I also like to dab on essential oils, such as sandalwood or lavender when I meditate. Some of my clients find they like using rose, geranium, patchouli or sweet orange. Before I begin to meditate, I light an incense stick and candle which I wave before the images on my altar. This ritual, known as "puja" in Sanskrit, is a moment where I acknowledge the divine presence in my life. You may wish to set an intention for your meditation, recite a prayer or offer your practice for the highest good.

There are several meditation apps available. "Insight Timer" is a free app and has many excellent meditations of all types ranging from five to sixty minutes.

Sylvia, a slender forty-one-year-old professional came to see one of the integrative doctors at Centre Spring and was recommended to me for Marma and Ayurveda. She had chronic candida (yeast) in her body that she had a hard time tackling. She had undergone various treatments but they provided only temporary relief. Frustrated and anxious, she was ready for a new approach. She also faced a lot of stress in her relationship with her partner. His drinking and lack of self-care rubbed off on her. She wanted to leave but could not find the courage or strength to do so. She also worked out of her house which made it that more difficult to make the break. In our initial visit, I recommended a daily meditation practice as well as a change in diet, and a few Ayurvedic herbs to address her candida. After a few energy healing sessions with me as well as following the herbal protocol and doctor's recommendations she began a process of reconnecting with herself in a renewed way. She began a twice-daily meditation practice. She not only began to heal her body but she gave her mind and spirit the space it needed to free herself from a toxic relationship. She did move out, and she learned that her candida only flared when she was faced with stress. She now has the tools to return to return to balance when she gets off track.

Vibrational Healing / Energy "Is" the Medicine

Vibrational medicine or energy healing was once dismissed as little more than "quackery." Some Western doctors may cling to such outmoded thinking, but for many doctors, energy healing is as essential a tool as a physician's stethoscope. Indeed, integrative physicians routinely refer patients for energy healing to remove energetic blocks in the form of trauma, grief, loss, sexual abuse or everyday stress and fatigue. Antidepressants are no longer the immediate go-to. This is certainly true in my own practice working with the well-known integrative doctor- Dr. Tasneem Bhatia.

Negative impressions collect over time in the human energy field much like a dirty attic collecting dust. Once this dust is removed, a person gains clarity, renewed vitality and can embark on a clear path to whole health. Rather than fixing symptoms, physicians, therapists, and healers are more and more often looking to address the root cause of physical symptoms. Many would say that the genesis of the ailment is almost always emotional: a dysfunctional marriage, unexpressed grief, the loss of a partner or pet, financial loss, work stress or children departing the home to live on their own or a child's inability to find her own way. Emotions that have been belittled or repressed can affect the body in various ways.

Haven't you experienced this yourself? You go to a mall and leave exhausted but head to a hiking trail with waterfalls and wildflowers and feel rejuvenated. That's energy. You sit with complaining people and feel drained but a few friends tell some jokes over dinner and everyone is uplifted. We experience energy every moment. We are drawn to certain relationships based upon energy.

But there's a deeper energy scientists are discovering, our perception and how it affects our chemistry. There is an exciting arena of research spearheaded by Dr. Bruce Lipton called Epigenetics that reveals that what we think and feel controls whether genes lean toward genetic predisposition of disease or change. This new paradigm goes beyond the human body as merely flesh, bones, joints, tissues and systems but rather sees the body as an energy field or bio-field of energy inclusive of things we cannot always see. Einstein said, "the field is the only reality." We are all part of a giant quantum energy field.

Ayurveda, the traditional holistic system of medicine from India, shows how the mind and the body are inextricably connected. A core premise is that nothing has more power to heal and transform the body than the mind.

Millennia before Western medicine, Ayurveda accurately described the human energy system and depicted, in detail, where the main energy centers in the body are located and how they work. Correcting imbalances in one's energy centers fine-tune a person's physical, emotional and mental health. Its vibrational toolkit can include color, sound or specific yoga postures. These energy centers, also known as "chakras," and the energy field surrounding the body can be seen using Kirlian and other special photographic techniques. Dr. Kelly Brogan writes in her book "A Mind of Your Own" that "energy medicine acknowledges that, fundamentally, our existence on this planet is attributable to unseen and poorly understood forces. Energy medicine does not rely on fallible beliefs about biology, the latest greatest paper, nor the reigning trend in combating disease. It relies simply on the gifts of healers who can unlock the body's healing potential, it puts us back in touch with our most fundamental driver- that chi, prana, or shakti or whatever word we use to describe that undeniable vital force that infuses our body with life and our mind with clarity and ease."

Can healing be so easy?

The earliest practitioners of Ayurveda understood that the body is made up of more than flesh, bones, muscles, tendons, and joints. They recognized and mapped, the body's vibrant pathways or energy channels that crisscross our nervous system and entire body. In traditional Chinese medicine, these are known as meridians. In Tibetan and Ayurvedic medicine, they are referred to as "nadis"- 72,000 of them.

Imagine a superhighway of channels that connect your entire being, an intricate spider web without beginning or end. A recent exhibit of Tibetan history at the Emory Museum, "Doorway to an Enlightened World," included a diagram drawn on parchment paper that illustrated this unique map of our physiology dating back thousands of years.

Jonathan Goldman, the author of "Healing Sounds: The Power of Harmonics," writes: "If parts of the body become imbalanced, they may be healed through projecting the proper and correct frequencies back into the body." Vibrational Medicine helps heal the energy body through therapies such as acupuncture and "Marma" — sensitive points in the body through which energy flows — to assess any imbalances or disharmonies. These areas can then be treated using the frequency from flower essences, sound, therapeutic essential oils, homeopathy, color, botanical herbs, and crystals. Each sound, color, crystal, or flower essence has a specific quality that is beneficial for a human organ, system or emotion.

When the flow of energy along these lines or "nadis" is impeded we feel sluggish or ill. But when our energy flows smoothly and freely, we experience vibrant health. Just as a river needs to flow freely within its banks, so too does the energy in our bodies if we are to feel clear and energetic. By shifting the bio-field we shift the body toward health and wellness. Since the mind and body are inseparable, Ayurveda prescribes many tools to lesson overthinking, obsessing over the past or future or other habits of mind that yank us out of the present moment.

The mind naturally finds poise and restful awareness through the practice of meditation, yoga, tai chi, qigong, gardening, dance, and creativity. (For more information, consult the chapter on Movement).

One form of energy medicine that is now mainstream is acupuncture. Many major insurance companies cover this ancient practice for pain relief, cessation of smoking, fertility, relieve headaches, fibromyalgia, fatigue, anxiety, osteoarthritis, menstrual cramps and more. Marma, the energy therapy of Ayurveda, works with the *chakras* to clear the emotional body, while acupuncture works with meridians to affect the physical body. Marma or Marmani are energy points that lie along the front and back of the body. When gently pressed the "prana" or life force in our bodies is stimulated releasing an inner pharmacy of natural chemicals such as serotonin, melatonin, oxytocin, and endorphins. Marma therapy relieves pain on all levels, increases energy flow, can be anti-aging and is restorative, calming and grounding. It increases a sense of overall well-being and has the unique benefit of being able to change one's perspective. Marma is only taught from teacher to student. Marma can also serve as a diagnostic tool where the practitioner can detect imbalances in the doshas, organs and bodily systems revealing valuable clues to healing. Both ancient systems of medicine recognize that each organ has an emotional, mental and physical component potentially storing past and present emotional trauma.

Some people find touch therapies reach deeper places in the unconscious than traditional talk therapy. Each approach has its benefits. Some touch therapists assert that their touch healing modalities access alternative pathways to the brain to change ingrained patterns.

Is raising my frequency essential to my health? Is low frequency an indication of poor health?

Researchers found that "the normal frequency range of the human body is between 62-68 MHz, but when it drops below that we can be subject to *dis-ease*. Cold symptoms appear at 58 MHz, flu symptoms at 57 MHz, candida at 55 MHz, Epstein bar at 52 MHz, cancer at 42 MHz. Simply put, if we can keep the body frequency high enough, and well oxygenated, we can remain disease free.

The body's trillion or so cells face formidable threats, and one of these comes from chemicals known as "free radicals." Antioxidants came to public attention in the 1990s, when scientists began to recognize their harmful effects. Antioxidants were seen as a way to eradicate the negative energy in our body and up the ante with oxygenating foods such as colorful fruits and vegetables. In addition to food; yoga, breath work, healthy relationships, exercise, chanting, meditation, and positive emotions these key ingredients serve to promote wellness and "good vibes."

How can I raise my frequency?

Here's a startling fact: essential oils are said to possess the highest frequency of any substance known to man. Ancient Egyptians used aromatic botanicals when preparing the deceased for mummification. Royal embalmers used botanicals such as cinnamon, and the resin from frankincense, myrrh, and ancient cedars and junipers to create essential oils.

Essential oils are easy to use and easy to carry— with no negative side effects. They are truly nature's gifts! A few drops of peppermint reduce stomach aches, improve mental focus and release tight muscles. A lemon essential oil can cleanse toxins, stimulate lymph drainage, and boost energy. Lavender oil reduces anxiety, improves sleep, and can alleviate burns and headaches.

Be sure to use high-quality, therapeutic grade oils that are organic, wildcrafted. Low-quality essential oils may be packaged with toxic ingredients that counteract the benefits of aromatherapy. What you apply to your skin goes directly into your bloodstream. When you use a high-quality oil, you will feel the results almost immediately within 15 minutes of application. Essential oils can benefit physical, mental and emotional health.

How do I use essential oils?

Aromatherapy, as it is known, is inhaling essential oils through a diffuser which is normally plugged into a wall socket. The best diffusers have a cool air mist (avoid heated diffusers which destroy the oils' essential properties). Simply add ten to fifteen drops of your favorite oil into the diffuser or use a combination of oils. There are also other effective ways to use essential oils such as adding oil to a bath. Just ten drops of therapeutic grade lavender, chamomile, rose or ylang ylang can be nourishing and healing after a busy day. A compress can easily be made by using warm distilled water- one cup with two to three drops of oil- dip a cloth in the water and apply. A couple of essential tips when it comes to oils :

- Always dilute them when using on the body, (such as with coconut oil, sesame, jojoba or sweet almond)
- Don't ingest them unless directed by the manufacturer and be cautious using them on pets and children. There are specific dilutions for children and pets that you can find with a little research.
- Don't apply oils to open wounds.

Here are a few recommendations for emotional healing:

- Add two drops with a carrier oil. Apply to the bottom of the feet, behind the neck or ears and on your wrists or add it to your bath or in your body massage oil.

For the following emotional states, use:

Mood Swings - Geranium
Anxiety - Lavender, frankincense, and sandalwood
Anger - Jasmine, rose, sage
Confidence - Jasmine and rosemary
Depression - lavender, juniper
Fear – ylang-ylang, frankincense
Grief/Loss – rose, ylang-ylang, neroli
Balance hormones - clary sage, holy basil
Grounding - vetiver
Fatigue (mental, emotional or physical) - nutmeg, juniper, geranium

Essential oils are highly effective for emotional healing as they affect the "limbic" part of the brain and promote awareness. Oils such as frankincense and sandalwood have high frequencies and are used for meditation. White Angelica can ward off negative energy and are often used by healers to protect their energy.

The best advice when using essential oils is to follow your nose. If you feel attracted to the scent of an essential oil, it is most likely good for you. Essential oils are a concentrated combination of a plant or tree's bark, leaves, and stems and hold the vibrational quality of that plant's intelligence. They somehow have a way of speaking to your highest need. Ask and you shall receive.

The American Holistic Nurses Association is now training RNs to use therapeutic grade essential oils, also known as aromatherapy, in a clinical setting.

I first began using essential oils when our children were young. I would apply a dab of Young Living Thieves oil to their feet before school and a bit of vetiver before sleep as a daily ritual. If they had a fever, I would mix peppermint and lavender with a carrier oil like sesame or sweet almond oil and apply it on their spine. The peppermint would help to break the fever without the use of over the counter meds. My son could soon return to class and playing tennis within a few days. After many years of competitive athletics, I once awoke with a ruptured disc. The therapist who came to my home used essential oils on my back — Roman chamomile, valor and lavender. After a few weeks of rest, oils and the use of a "tens machine," my back healed, much to the surprise of my orthopedist. He was curious what I had done to heal so quickly.

Ten oils I recommend you start with are:

Lavender, peppermint or spearmint, eucalyptus, lemon, orange, rosemary, ylang-ylang, sandalwood, geranium, and holy basil.

The following companies sell high-quality essential oils- Young Living(Utah), Mountain Rose (Oregon), Nature's Gifts (Tennessee). Bulk Apothecary also has organic oils providing more competitive pricing. Diffusers can be purchased through any of these companies.

Color

I like red, you may prefer blue or someone else loves green. So, what's in a color? Just like the colors of the rainbow, each color contains a vibratory frequency, much as musical notes. We know that red means stop and green means go, black is generally worn at funerals and white at weddings. But there are more profound ways colors affect our emotions. Rudolf Steiner, the Austrian founder of the esoteric spiritual movement known as anthroposophy and Waldorf schools, advocated painting each classroom a different color depending on the developmental age of the child. For example, the kindergarten was painted in peachy tones representing the softness of the soul. He found this soothed the often out of control energy of young children.

Orange or ginger is often recommended on the walls in a dining area to help digestion, while blue or lavender for a room promotes a good night's sleep. Green fosters calm, while red can be stimulating.

The body's subtle energy system mirrors the rainbow, starting from the root chakra and up to the crown, in a spectrum of red, orange, yellow, green, blue, indigo and violet.

Colored light therapy, known as chromotherapy, is used in Europe to heal various physical conditions. Wrapping a cup of water in colored tissue paper and setting it under the sunlight can infuse it with colored light. In India, while completing my clinical training in Ayurveda, I witnessed Dr. Lad recommend selected patient's wrap a glass of water with green tissue paper- set it on the window sill for an hour and then drink it to absorb the vibrations of light. Green was chosen to reduce stress and anxiety.

We are continuously encouraged to eat "colorful" food so we can receive the "full spectrum" of light into our bodies, thereby raising our oxygen intake and frequency.

When we spend time in nature we bathe our bodies in the full spectrum of colored light nourishing us on all levels. The Vitamin D benefits are essential for over 300 bodily functions including the absorption of other minerals such as magnesium.

Sound

The pitter-patter of falling rain. The sound of a babbling brook. The crackling of burning logs. Why is it certain sounds soothe us and help us relax or fall asleep?

Of course, the opposite is also true. Nails on a blackboard. A crying baby. A high-pitched shriek. For most of us, such sounds are grating and irritating.

From firsthand experience, we grasp the power of sound to affect us. Each of us is sensitive to a person's tone of voice and hear and feels the difference between someone barking, "Come here!" versus a hushed, sweet invitation to "Come here."

While we experience sounds as pleasant or unpleasant, we may fail to recognize the power of sound to heal. Specific sounds, be it a gong, singing bowl, mantras, chants or music all share a vibratory quality or frequency that can heal and soothe the body and mind.

In our everyday lives, consciously or not, we comfort ourselves with sound. Children often sing when they play. Some adults—and dwarves—whistle or hum while they work. Teens may blast loud music to rouse themselves awake.

There's nothing New Age about using sound for healing, it's as old as the pyramids. Many creation stories began with a sonorous event. In the ancient Vedic scriptures of India, the cosmos is birthed from the sound *Aum* (Om). The Gospel of John opens with the verse: "In the beginning was the Word...." The world's great cathedrals, mosques, and temples were often built to magnify the power of sound, be it from an organ, a cantor or the voices from a choir.

A Gregorian choir, a muezzin perched in a minaret calling the faithful to prayer or the choral singing of the Maori of New Zealand, every culture and faith tradition has its version of sacred song. It's widely acknowledged across history, region, and tradition that sound can soothe the soul.

The Greek philosopher, Pythagoras of Samos, was said to have used therapeutic music to treat physical as well as emotional maladies. Ancient Aztecs texts refer to a Creator who "sang the world into existence."

It's been said that "Vibrations resulting from devotional singing lead to attunement with the Cosmic Vibration or the Word." The Sufi master, Hazrat Inayat Khan, went so far as to say: "What makes us feel drawn to music is that our whole being is music; our mind and body, the nature in which we live, the nature which has made us, all that is beneath and around us, it is all music."

The 14th-century Sufi poet Hafiz exclaimed, "People say that the soul, on hearing the song of creation, entered the body, but, in reality, the soul itself was the song."

In short, when the mind is quiet, the soul hears. Listening to or playing sacred music empowers the mind to perceive and release illusions of isolation, fear, and suffering. Some spiritual teachers, view sound, not gravity, as the primary organizing force of all matter in the early Universe.

If sound was the trigger for life, it should not be a surprise that sound can support and heal life. There's growing interest in using sound frequency to boost human health, and medical studies back it up. In "The Science Behind Healing with Sound," writer Kathryn Drury Wagner cites the groundbreaking work of biophysicist Gerald Oster. In the 1970s, Oster "showed that when a tone is played in one ear and a slightly different tone is played in the other ear, the difference causes the brain to create a third, internal tone, called a binaural beat. The theory is that this syncs the brain waves in both hemispheres, a process dubbed "brain-wave entrainment."

Clinical studies have shown that brain-wave entrainment is an effective tool to use on cognitive functioning deficits, stress, pain, headaches, premenstrual syndrome as well as behavioral issues. Some neuro-acoustic researchers and healers say that certain sounds can boost immunity and treat insomnia.

Some practitioners refer to the potential of sound to heal as "frequency medicine."

How does it work?

Sound causes shifts in our brain wave state by something called entrainment. Entrainment synchronizes our fluctuating brainwaves by providing a stable frequency which our brain waves attune to. By using rhythm and frequency our brain waves move from normal waking consciousness to "alpha," a relaxed consciousness or "theta," a deep meditative state. One modality to achieve this is sound baths. Sound affects both the physical and subtle body and helps to open energetic pathways. As a result, energy blocks are removed and our life force flows more freely. It's the vibration itself that opens energetic pathways and moves stagnant *qi*.

Scientists and doctors may not use those terms or explain the power of sound healing in such terms, nonetheless many recognize its benefits of sound to help us sleep, reduce stress or bolster our immune system.

How can sound be used?

In the Jewish tradition, it is considered a commandment to listen to the sound of the *shofar* (ram's horn) on the High Holidays during the month of Elul, September. The shofar played in synagogues on Rosh Hashanah, the Jewish New Year, is viewed as an "alarm" a signal for the soul to turn within. I feel its sound reverberate down the spine.

While more and more healers and yoga studios offer "sound baths" and various other sound healing rituals, the bottom line is while those are beneficial and a great introduction to the power of sound healing, you don't need a degree or expensive equipment to experience its benefits. Indeed, the very sound of your own voice may prove to be the most powerful healing tool. Sing in the shower. Hum while you walk. I'm struck when watching professional tennis when players release a powerful sound as they return a serve.

Studies show that even a short bout of singing can increase immunoglobulin A, an antibody. Apart from prepping for karaoke, *The Voice* or the release of your next YouTube video, singing is good for your health. So too is singing with others, be it in the front seat of your car while on a drive with a friend or with a choir.

If human voices don't do the trick for you, consider listening to the sound of animals. Dolphins use sound to signal each other. Their clicks or the song of whales are said to relax the body and mind.

The significance of sound is perceived even before we are born. Dr. Alfred A. Tomatis, a French sound researcher, found that a mother's state of mind during her pregnancy has a significant impact on the child. When an expectant mother listens to soothing sounds during her pregnancy, the benefits are passed on to the fetus.

Sound healing advocates say that listening to percussive instruments like gongs, Tibetan singing bowls, and tuning forks reduce stress and place the listener in a meditative state. Practitioners use sound healing as an alternative treatment for anxiety, chronic pain, sleep disorders and PTSD.

What are tuning forks?

Tuning forks look like a two-pronged fork and, when struck, resonate sound that increases energy flow and grounds the breath. When you strike a tuning fork, it causes the air around the fork to vibrate, sending out vibrating impulses through the air. Originally used to tune musical instruments, healers use them to help relieve stress, reduce inflammation, open the breath or increase oxygen and energy flow. Tuning forks can be applied to almost any area of the body and are often used in concert with other modalities such as Marma, Massage, Shiatsu or Cranial-Sacral.

Because the body is made up of more than 70% water, sound easily conducts through its channels. I've been impressed with the "Ohm Therapeutics" tuning forks, which are said to be tuned to the earth's vibration around the sun. I find the earth tone sound vibration of *Aum* deeply relaxing, grounding and energizing.

Research by Dr. John Beaulieu on sound healing found that tuning forks also have the ability to release nitric oxide in the body, a pain-modulating substance that can reduce inflammation, improve digestion, vascular health, and immune function while improving energy, reducing stress and depression.

Tuning forks can easily be used at home. It's easy to experiment on oneself or a friend. Start with the top of the head, the center of the forehead, the back of the neck, the center of the chest, center of the abdomen at the belly button, middle of the upper thigh, knee, calf, and bottom of the feet. They are easy to use, simply tap the fork on the rubber stand it comes with and hold the base with your thumb and forefinger without touching the two prongs. This sequence can be done daily. It is incredibly refreshing, energizing, relaxing and grounding all at once. You can start your day with this sequence before or after meditation.

We can use sound to uplift us, foster calm, or reset the tone within ourselves or in our environment to help us better meet our daily work and responsibilities.

Quality tuning forks are available at www.soundhealingtools. com.

Another method of working with sound is through learning about the distinct sacred sounds or mantras associated with each of the seven chakras. Chakras have both distinct colors and sounds or mantras that can heal that energy center. One can easily tune the chakras with these syllables by holding them in your awareness and repeating them three times. You may wish to address the specific chakra region where you are feeling pain or discomfort. For example, if you have digestive issues you can choose the sound "Ram" and repeat it three times while sitting or lying down allowing the sound to vibrate in the area around your abdomen or solar plexus. If you have lower back pain you may use the sound "Lam" and repeat it three times while placing your awareness on the lower back. The "m" sound at the end of these tones should be exaggerated such as "mmmmmm."

The CD "Toning the Chakras" with Joy Gardner Gordon is one I highly recommend. You can purchase it at www.highvibrations. net. The images on the CD were taken before and after toning the chakras. The colors of the aura changed dramatically from dull, depleted and exhausted to relaxed, centered and radiant. It's fascinating to see.

Chanting

Singer and author, Durga Das, says "kirtan" is a means to praise the divine or "that which is exalted." Its Sanskrit root means "to cut through," he says, so kirtan is also "a practice for cutting through the idea of separation, for connecting to our hearts and connecting to the moment through sound."

Kirtan derives from India's ancient call-and-response form of chanting the names of a myriad of gods and goddesses that are central to religions such as Hinduism and Sikhism as well as the names of revered gurus. Grammy-nominated *kirtan* singer Krishna Das, tells Kripalu that we honor a space, a presence, a feeling. These names [of Hindu deities] are the names of that place inside of us that is love, pure being, pure awareness, pure joy." Kirtan, says Krishna Das—along with other forms of mantra practice, such as seated meditation—help us uncover that place inside of us.

In her book, "Courage and Contentment," Siddha Yoga meditation master, Gurumayi Chidvilasananda, writes, "The joy of chanting unfurls the inner world." Chanting has the power to dissolve our worries, still the mind for meditation and bring lightheartedness. Sound penetrates the emotional body where the root cause of many physical symptoms and disease begins.

While most *kirtan* chants last anywhere from 30 minutes to an hour, some can continue for a full week or more. The deeper one plunges into the chant, the more the grip of our small ego fades and the more connected we feel with our deepest Self. While the tradition is ancient, the practice has been embraced and at times reinvented in the West where some *kirtan* singers blend traditional *kirtan* with electronica and other musical genres.

Kirtan can also be enjoyed solo. *Kirtan* singers from Krishna Das to Jai Uttal and Deva Premal all have dozens of CDs that one can chant along with while walking, driving, cooking or before sitting to meditate.

I'm a great lover of *kirtan* and at my graduation from an Ayurveda training course in India a well-known Indian tabla player performed for us. When I took his picture all that showed up on the camera was swirling colors of light. I checked to confirm my camera was working just fine and when I showed him the photo, he smiled.

Singing Bowls

Tibetan singing bowls have been used for healing and meditation for thousands of years. You may have heard one at the end of your hatha yoga class as a prelude to the "Aum" chant. Their soothing notes and frequencies create a range of sound to restore the body's harmony. Like a musical instrument that is out of tune, stress, anxiety, depression, and grief can pull us out of alignment. The sound of singing bowls, whether live or recorded, can have profound benefits to our sympathetic and parasympathetic nervous systems. Many yoga studios now hold concerts with Tibetan bowls.

Of course, one of the most potent and profound sounds is our very own inner voice, whether you refer to it as the Self or God. It's available to dial into anytime if we simply create a "gap" or pause in our consciousness to make space to hear.

This process of inner listening puts us in a space whereby the mind stills and the body relaxes. In this state, the mind is moved into a present-time reality where the sacred vibration of harmony (Aum, Amen, or Cosmic Vibration) is least distorted and the mind is quiet enough to both witness and remember the Song of the Self. We then feel identified with an inner awareness of "I AM," or the Divinity within.

Sacred sounds are simply tools that help us to praise the divine and remember our divine nature.

Gemstones

To begin with, gemstones are just plain stunning. Gemstones and crystals were forged millions of years ago during the earliest days of earth's formation. Pharaohs, emperors, and queens have adorned themselves with precious gems in their crowns, robes, and jewelry. Warriors, shamans, and priests have worn them as talismans or amulets.

Gems and minerals formed when molten rock, or magma, cools. These precious gifts from the Earth have been prized across cultures and history. At first glance, they may appear as nothing more than an ordinary rock. It's only when they are cut and polished that they obtain the brilliance and luster that gives them their value.

While we give the gift of a diamond, ruby, sapphire or emerald to commemorate life's most valued events—minerals and gems are key components in many cutting-edge technologies from lasers to computers to smartphones.

It's no wonder, many have come to embrace gemstones and crystals and their vibratory power as a source of healing and protection. Gems are said to transmit, reflect, store light and receive and emit energy. When placed directly on your body, they are believed to have a powerful vibratory effect that surges from the crystal to you.

Scientifically speaking, there is no evidence that crystal healing can be used to cure disease, yet so many people find that simply being in the presence or holding a crystal or gemstone, unleashes a sense of calm or positive energy. While popular at spas, New Age bookstores and with many healers, ancient cultures in China, Egypt, Greece and Latin America also embraced gemstones as conduits for protection and healing.

How it's supposed to work

Modern crystal healing is based on traditional concepts borrowed from Asian cultures, notably the Chinese concept of qi, life energy, and the Hindu and Buddhist concept of chakras, which are energy centers in the subtle body.

In many cultures, people carry gemstones on their bodies or place them around their home, even under a pillow to ward off ill health or ill fortune. If you subscribe to the premise that everything in existence is imbued with the intelligence of Universal Consciousness—call it creative energy, vibration, or life force—this energy manifests in myriad forms in nature.

In crystal healing, each gemstone is believed to be beneficial for a specific part of the body. Amethyst, for example, benefits the intestines; green aventurine helps the heart; yellow topaz sharpens mental clarity.

During a treatment session, a crystal healer may place various stones or crystals on your body at specific chakra points, most often above the head, on the forehead, on the throat, on the chest, on the stomach, on the gut, or legs. I use them in my Marma sessions.

Turquoise was a highly-prized gem of the Aztecs, the Persians, Tibetans and Native Americans. The healing powers of turquoise can benefit the whole body, with a particular ability to heal ailments of the immune, respiratory, waste and skeletal systems. It's also said to promote qualities of love, strength, and affection.

Amber is highly effective for controlling the pain of rheumatism, arthritis, and aching muscles and joints. Baltic Amber has also been used as an anti-anxiety remedy and is said to lessen fatigue, weariness, headaches, and problems affecting the neck and throat areas. Amber can be worn as a ring or as a bracelet. It affects the solar plexus chakra increasing self-esteem, self-confidence. It also protects one from the negative effects of radiation.

Amethyst, a purple translucent stone, helps to open the crown chakra, affecting the pineal and pituitary glands. It's also considered helpful to soothe headaches and balance blood sugar. Experiment by placing an amethyst stone at the head of the bed or on a night table.

Rose Quartz is a rose-pink variety of Quartz. Rose quartz is the stone of universal love and compassion. It restores trust and harmony in relationships, encouraging unconditional love. Rose quartz purifies and opens the heart at all levels to promote love, self-love, friendship, deep inner healing and feelings of peace. It can be worn as a pendant or by putting a stone in your meditation area or bedroom near your pillow. Try taking an afternoon pause by resting for five minutes with a rose quartz on the heart chakra. It can feel transforming.

For female hormonal imbalances, especially hot flashes, mother of pearl can be used around the neck or as a ring on the left pinky finger, according to Ayurveda. Its cooling nature affects hyperacidity and can reduce inflammation.

Jade Green is said to be good for health, and to attract wealth, longevity, and happiness, according to Chinese Medicine. It benefits the lungs, heart, immune and thymus.

Lapis, a deep blue stone, can be worn around the neck to improve communication and affect the thyroid. It is also a stone of protection that may be worn to guard against psychic attacks. Lapis Lazuli quickly releases stress, bringing deep peace. It brings harmony and deep inner self-knowledge.

Citrine, a yellow-orange stone, has a warm and sunny vibration that can assist with alleviating anxiety, due to its energies of optimism and joy. Citrine is a great ally for activating the imagination and channeling negative emotions into creative pursuits, thereby sparking a more positive outlook. Citrine is also known to assist in the release of repressed anger, which can often be a hidden cause of anxiety.

Let's not forget the diamond—a girl's best friend. High in vibrational energy, diamonds are believed to strengthen one's connection to divine consciousness. Interesting how diamonds are viewed as the gem of choice for a wedding ring, perhaps due to its potent energy of union.

Diamonds are recommended for people seeking relief from grief and depression! It also enhances one's clarity, acuity, and memory. It is also a helpful gemstone for individuals with a short-temper.

Gems, crystals, and minerals are excellent tools for personal growth.

Though forged by molten rock, intense pressure or physical forces like ice, wind, and water, you will still need to take care of your gemstones. Wash them in salt water when you get them and after using them on other people. If no water is at hand, hold them in your hand, and say a prayer.

There are no scientific studies so far that validate the claims of the healing power of gemstones. Many may dismiss their benefits as nothing more than a placebo effect, though it's impossible to deny the powerful results experienced by people from around the globe.

Allow your heart to gravitate to the stones that speak to you. For high-quality gems visit a jewelry store or gemologist. There's a variety of sizes, colors, shapes to choose from.

Remember, when using any modality considered "alternative" or invalidated by science and medicine, do not ignore the advice of your physician. However, there's no harm in experimenting with gemstones and discovering how or if it can benefit your health, mood or inner state. Your body needs tuning like a fine musical instrument. Gemstones and crystals can help you tune into emotional well-being and health.

Nutrition / How Food Nourishes the Body and Spirit

" S cientists have found that rituals performed around food actually influence the way the food is enjoyed," writes Catherine Saint Louis and Vijay Singh, in *The New York Times* article, "Rituals Make Your Own Food More Flavorful." "We all have our food rituals -- from splitting apart the Oreo cookie to folding a pizza slice." And we know from experience how much better a birthday cake tastes when you've been serenaded by friends before you dig in. We each delight in our own idiosyncratic food rituals, many from childhood, be it licking the sides of an ice cream cone before it melts or twirling spaghetti onto a fork before taking a big bite.

Far more often than we acknowledge, our meals are not only devoid of ritual, but mechanical, even joyless. We scarf down a burger while stalled in traffic, inhale microwaved dinners while mindlessly watching television or treat health bars as if they were the equivalent of a wholesome, nutritious meal.

It turns out that taking pleasure in food and receiving optimal nourishment from food, are linked.

Of course, our "excuses" to avoid taking the time to prepare, share or enjoy a meal are legion: "Who has time?" "Healthy, organic food is crazy expensive" or "I can't be bothered to go to all the fuss when it's just me eating alone."

Michael Pollan, the author of numerous bestselling books about food and food culture and politics, is known for his simple, pithy advice to: "Eat food. Not too much. Mostly plants."

But Pollan writes not only about what to eat, but how we eat.

"The French paradox," he writes, "is that they have better heart health than we do despite being a cheese-eating, wine-swilling, foisgras gobbling people. The American paradox is we are a people who worry unreasonably about dietary health yet have the worst diet in the world."

What are some simple ways we can shift our approach to how we eat so it is nourishing, fun and good for our digestion?

Step One – Eat slowly

The benefits of slow eating include better digestion, better hydration, greater weight loss or weight maintenance as well as more satisfaction. Eating quickly, however, contributes to poor digestion, increased weight gain and lower satisfaction. That about sums it up.

More than 10 percent of the world's population is now obese. That translates to nearly 604 million adults worldwide who are obese and 108 million children, according to a 2017 study compiled by the Institute for Health Metrics and Evaluation at the University of Washington.

The United States had the dubious distinction of having the largest increase in percentile jump in obesity of any country, a gain of 16 percentage points to 26.5 percent of the overall population.

With the weight gain came a sharp spike in heart disease, diabetes, kidney disease.

What can you do?

In addition to diet and exercise, simply chewing your food is an excellent start. Key to this is bringing your full attention to the food you are eating and chewing it until it's mush or the consistency of baby food. That means you will first need to turn off *NCIS, Sunday Night Football* or *The Big Bang Theory.*

Before that first bite, you can transform the rote act of eating into a ritual or moment of thanks. Say a prayer to God or to the farmer who grew the food, the cook who prepared it or the people sitting with you at the table. If your brain is plugged into reading *People Magazine*, answering texts or absorbed in a YouTube video, you're far less likely to remember to eat slowly, chew or relax.

We actually digest food better when the act of eating commands our full attention. If you live alone, consider creating a weekly ritual where a friend or group of friends get together to share a meal. If you live with a partner or have kids, make it a point to designate a few nights in the week where you sit down together to break bread. Prepare food together. Get the kids involved. Create your own food rituals. This isn't about feeling pressure to be the "perfect" host or prepare the perfect gourmet meal, this is about enjoying good food and good company.

Step Two – Eat food (Not processed, food-like substances)

One thing I often shared with our children growing up was "If it doesn't grow, don't eat it." Food writer, Michael Pollan has his own version: "If it doesn't rot don't eat it." The longer the ingredient list on the back of a box, the further it is from the soil. Although our pantry wasn't filled with sugary or salty snacks children often crave, my children's friends nonetheless struck me as taking genuine pleasure in snacking on the fresh fruit that was always set out on the center island of our kitchen, the homemade guacamole with organic chips or the nightly dinners prepared with fresh food from our garden.

Despite the hectic schedule of the kids' afterschool tennis and music lessons, we made it a priority to have fresh food and healthy snacks on hand. Like many families, we also had our rituals, including eating out at a great family-owned Chinese restaurant in town that was our go-to spot after the kids' games.

While the center aisles of grocery stores remain filled with processed foods, farmer's markets are now more common, and more and more supermarkets stock locally-grown foods. I advise my clients here in Atlanta to shop for produce that is grown in Georgia, Alabama, Tennessee or North Carolina rather than from Mexico, Peru or even California, since it has been shipped 1600 miles. The best solution of all is to grow food in your garden. I've found children love gardening: the digging in the dirt to the tall pea poles, which can be prolific and their giant sunflowers or potted zucchini plants.

The joy of cooking is simply an abstract and foreign concept to many of us. Lots of us live on the usual fare: hamburger Mondays, take-out Tuesdays or fish-stick Fridays. There may well be a link in the rise in popularity of cooking shows and the decline of people's ability to cook. The thing is, you don't have to be a professional chef for cooking to be imaginative, healthful and fun.

Marvel at the colors of nature and select foods from the full color spectrum. Be bold! Consider trying new veggies and new recipes. Let your children pick produce that they're curious to eat.

The spectrum of natural color in fresh produce isn't only beautiful, it also happens to be a useful indicator of the many health benefits of fresh, plant-based foods. The deep greens, vibrant reds, deep purples, bright oranges & yellows that we see in widely available foods provide far more than just "a rainbow" of colors. Each pack its own distinct beneficial nutrients.

Slow Food is a grassroots organization founded by Carlo Petrini in Italy in 1986. It has since spread worldwide and continues to advocate for affordable, quality, flavorsome and healthy food grown whose production does not harm the environment. To learn more about the organization, visit *www.slowfoodusa.org*. The group also works to preserve, defend regional traditions, gastronomic pleasure and a slow pace of life.

For over 25 years, Community Supported Agriculture has become a popular way for consumers to buy local, seasonal food directly from a local farmer. The farmer usually offers a basket of food for the week (of whatever is in season). For more information, *visit www.localharvest.org.*

Step Three – Go Alkaline

In "Tired of Feeling the Burn? Low-Acid Diet May Help," Tara Parker-Pope, a *The New York Times* wellness columnist, writes: "Stomach acid has long been blamed for acid reflux, heartburn, and other ills. But now some experts are starting to think that the problems may lie not just in the acid coming up from the stomach but in the food going down."

Indeed! The bottom line when it comes to food is that the American diet is primarily acidic. Imbalance and disease can set in when the body is dealing with too many acid-forming foods. In an acid environment, the body begins to deplete its alkaline resources and becomes more susceptible to disease and a compromised immune system. Acid forming foods can create the perfect storm for a host of other diseases as well as be the culprit for inflammation. Packaged and processed foods, as well as breads, pasta, alcohol, coffee, are all examples of acid-forming foods and beverages. Even breads labeled "whole wheat" are acidic let alone prescription drugs that have an acidic effect on the body. You may not want to give up your coffee but by simply adding cardamom and a pinch of cinnamon you can alter the pH.

Maintaining a balance of 80 percent alkaline foods and 20 percent acidic foods is considered ideal. Some studies find that regulating your body's acid/alkaline chemistry and can result in weight loss, increased stamina and strength, and a stronger immune system.

What can we do to move toward an alkaline eco inner environment?

Here are five simple tips from a holistic health approach:

1. Consume at least one or two servings daily of dark leafy greens slightly cooked.
2. Cook with ghee. Ghee is clarified butter. It is good for lactose intolerant people and is alkalizing. Ghee builds the immune system, strengthens the body and according to Ayurvedic medicine has anti-aging properties.
3. Consume these alkalizing fruits: avocados, pears, peaches, cherries, apples, all types of melon, dates, papayas, figs and red grapes. Some dairy products are alkaline, such as buttermilk, raw milk, plain yogurt (homemade) and acidophilus milk. Amaranth and quinoa are alkalizing grains. Almonds, chestnuts and fresh coconut are all alkalizing. Other alkaline foods include raw honey, kelp, green tea and egg yolks. Lentils, mung beans and vegetables are also alkalizing. Regular shots of wheatgrass, spirulina or chlorella are also beneficial and very worthwhile to include in your daily diet. They have been called "superfoods" because they are packed with vital nutrients.

Just as there is no one food or nutrient that provides everything we need, likewise, no single color provides all the necessary nutritional power. That is the premise of Chris Woollams' book, "The Rainbow Diet." Professor Ralph Stewart of Auckland City Hospital, New Zealand, has demonstrated that adherence to the Rainbow Diet greatly reduces heart attack, stroke and cardiovascular risk.

A former Oxford University Biochemist, Woollams writes that he was struck by the study's finding that it was more beneficial to "be positive and to tell people to eat a Rainbow Diet than it was to tell them to avoid certain foods."

Step Four — Ayurveda to the Rescue

From the Scarsdale Diet to the Beverly Hills Diet—not to mention, the Atkins, South Beach, Raw Food, Zone or Paleo diet—it's understandable that women and men today are confused about what to eat. We've been bombarded with exercise and food models that just don't stand up or don't address our individual needs.

Ayurveda, which originated in India over 5000 years ago, offers an individualized approach to health that makes it unique and applicable in our modern world. The Chopra Center explains that "The two main guiding principles of Ayurveda are 1) the mind and the body are inextricably connected, and 2) nothing has more power to heal and transform the body than the mind. Freedom from illness depends upon expanding our own awareness." Ayurveda understood long before modern medicine that what we eat affects our mind and emotions.

Ayurveda promotes a life close to nature—your own nature and the environment—and advocates a lifestyle that is in harmony with the seasons and ultimately provides a pathway to knowing the essence of your being and full potential. Preventing illness is a hallmark of Ayurveda and is done through paying close attention to one's right thinking, diet, lifestyle and the use of herbs and foods to balance health.

From an Ayurvedic perspective, health includes feeling content, joyous, bright and tranquil.

Health is not a one-size-fits-all approach.

Each person has a unique constitution or mind-body type they are born with, known in Ayurveda as one's *dosha*. Any movement away from that constitution creates health imbalances. If such imbalances are not addressed, then disease sets in.

When an Ayurvedic specialist looks at the tongue and pulse, these imbalances can be determined and corrected through specific herbs, essential oils, foods, gemstones, and lifestyle. The National Ayurvedic Medical Association provides trained practitioners around the country. www.ayurvedanama.org.

Since one's health is not static, Ayurveda can address the many changes and influences both inside and outside that affect our lives.

How can Ayurvedic nutrition principles help me feel strong, fit and vibrant?

The first step is to take a *dosha* quiz to determine your mind/body type. You can visit www.gedaliahhealingarts.com/services to take the quiz. Each of us are born with the influence of a primary or dual combination of nature's elements: ether, air, fire, water and earth. Each of the *doshas*—*vata*, *pitta*, and *kapha*—have specific mental, emotional and physical characteristics. These are not necessarily good or bad, they are simply tendencies. For instance, a person who is *vata* often has a tendency toward being cold, a slim boney physique, weak digestion often leading to constipation, and a creative mind which can easily get out of balance with too much movement or distraction. They are prone to anxiety, worry, arthritis, and nervous disorders. My colleague Anna Russ a biologist and teacher of Ayurveda, likens a person with a *vata* constitution to a greyhound dog.

A *pitta* dominant person is of medium build with a sharp intellect and competitive spirit—they are usually warm-blooded— and possess a strong digestion and have an affinity toward jealousy, attachment, and overwork. They are prone to rashes and diarrhea and overheating in summer. They can be compared to a German Shepherd.

A *kapha* person is usually larger boned, has tendencies toward sluggishness and procrastination, and are often very loving and grounded by nature. They need stimulation and invigorating activities to find balance such as biking, running or hot yoga. The dog analogy for a *kapha* person is a St. Bernard.

To achieve balance and more vibrant health, a *vata* person requires: warming foods, oils and a stabilized routine to reduce stress and anxiety. Calming exercise such as gentle yoga or tai chi. Grounding activities might include painting, working with clay, drawing or meditation.

To find balance, a *pitta* person benefits from: cooling foods, chill time, tai chi, doing work as service and being near water.

For a *kapha* person, balance is found through; stimulating pungent foods, vigorous exercise, and avoiding sweets for emotional comfort.

Knowing your *dosha* can be a helpful guide. Doshas can change with the seasons and one's age so it's best to consult with an Ayurvedic Specialist or doctor to determine your current state of health.

In Ayurveda, there are six tastes or *rasas*: sweet, sour, salty, bitter, pungent, and astringent. Ayurveda recommends including each of the tastes by the end of your day in your food. In a perfect world, they would be present in each meal.

According to Ayurveda, the best way to know if a food is good for you is one that you can easily digest. That means an absence of gas, bloating, acid reflux, cramps or irritable bowel. A hearty vegetable soup with veggies in season is an easy quick meal(s) for cooks and non-cooks to get the most nutrients from one single dish.

Warm, cooked, slightly oily foods are recommended for all three doshas. This sounds contrary to the raw food diets. According to Ayurveda, if a person has strong digestion they can eat raw foods, however, when one is weak and their immune system is compromised, warm, cooked food is suggested. What is the best food for me to eat? One that I can easily digest.

Here are a few basic Ayurvedic dietary principles:

- Aim to eat fruit alone in the morning or afternoon by itself.
- Your largest meal should be at lunch.
- Drink warm water or water at room temperature. Avoid cold, iced drinks and microwaved, leftover or packaged foods.
- Add turmeric, coriander, ginger, and garlic in your food.
- Lastly, and importantly, eat only when you are happy.

If you just take the best from this approach rather than looking at it as a "diet" you will find simple gems to enhance your health.

By listening to your body, eating foods you digest well, staying close to nature, and by eating in moderation you are paving your own road toward optimal health rather than feeling enslaved by prescription drugs.

An Ayurvedic proverb says" When diet is incorrect, medicine is of no use- when diet is correct, medicine is of no need".

How does Chinese medicine approach nutrition?

Like Ayurveda, Chinese medicine refers a person to pay close attention to their digestion avoiding the "designer diet" approach. The simple idea of listening to your body is at the heart of TCM approach.

An excellent resource about Chinese medicine is Paul Pitchford's *Healing with Whole Foods*. It is considered the bible of Traditional Chinese Medicine's approach to nutrition. You can look up the properties of specific foods along with recipes for foods. The book also addresses seasonal and environmental connections according to the

TCM philosophy, organ systems, disease syndromes, and recommendations for chronic imbalances.

Can I benefit from a Mediterranean diet?

A Mediterranean diet has been highly promoted by heart specialist Dr. Dean Ornish. Ornish found that when his patients switched to whole grains, vegetables, fruits and lean proteins as their main diet, it reversed the progression of heart disease. Due to his research at the Preventative Medicine Research Institute, in Sausalito, CA, Dr. Ornish began training physicians and other health professionals at eight hospitals throughout the country to demonstrate his results. Yes, there are helpful lessons to be gleaned from those who have lived the longest and the healthiest lives on our planet.

Some key components of a Mediterranean diet are:

1. Use olive oil as a main source of fat and throw out the margarine or fake butter.
2. Eliminate simple carbs such as white flour, white sugar and replace them with whole grains such as quinoa, barley, buckwheat, millet and brown rice.
3. Avoid over-consumption of red meat and instead consume lean proteins such as wild fish, turkey, and chicken.
4. Eat fruit as a snack.
5. Eat as many vegetables as you like.
6. Snack on raw nuts and seeds.

The best practices from these approaches provide anti-inflammatory foods, a lifestyle close to nature and most of all the self-care, and self-nourishment that ultimately leads to feeling wholesome and vibrant.

Betty, a forty-two-year-old working woman came to the practice Centre Spring MD. after struggling with health issues (digestive problems and joint pain) brought on by grief and stress. Betty learned her Ayurvedic energy type after a pulse evaluation and began making simple changes to her diet and lifestyle such as eating warm, cooked foods, simple digestible meals, and with oiling her body with recommended essential oils. She said, "It is so refreshing to have someone give me helpful suggestions of things "to do" rather than a list of things "not to do"." In just a few weeks I have seen a significant reduction in pain, am sleeping better and have even lost weight! I am very grateful to have found a new way of looking at health."

The Joy of Movement

In many shamanic societies, if you came to a shaman or medicine person complaining of being disheartened, dispirited, or depressed, they would ask one of four questions.
When did you stop dancing?
When did you stop singing?
When did you stop being enchanted by stories?

—Gabrielle Roth, an American dancer and musician

*I*n *Brain, Body & Being: Five Secrets for Achieving Authentic Health & Happiness,* Jay Kumar, a professor of cognitive science and happiness studies at Chapman University, cites a 20-year study published in the *New England Journal of Medicine* about the powerful link between dance and physical and cognitive health. "The long-term study of senior citizens set out to ascertain if physical activities and cognitive activities, such as reading, doing crossword puzzles, writing or playing a musical instrument diminished the risk of Alzheimer's disease. What they found was stunning.

"Of all the activities, both cognitive and physical, dancing had the highest ability to reduce the risk of dementia and Alzheimer's disease. How much so? People who reported to dance regularly had a 76% reduced chance of cognitive impairment!"

What did the scientists conclude? That dancing has one thing that differentiates it from other activities in their study. "Dancing uses more areas of our brain's memory and learning centers than other activities.

When we dance, we simultaneously integrate several brain functions: movement, emotion, music, thinking, sight, touch, and hearing.

"In essence, people who dance are building a bigger 'cognitive reserve' in their brains than those who don't. The more cognitive capital we accumulate, the more our brains remain healthy and strong.

The benefits of dancing are extensive and impressive:

- An effective antidote to stress and depression, dancing regulates our mood by stimulating the hippocampus and releases endorphins.
- Dancing doubles the brain's blood and oxygen levels.
- In addition to dancing's short-term benefits for regulating our mood and emotions, it's the long-term impact of dance on memory and brain health that is garnering even more attention.

I've seen the truth of this in my own life and witnessed the transformational power of movement among my friends, clients, and neighbors. Cleo, an 87-year-old, was a lithe Scandinavian blonde who I met while living in Santa Rosa California. She took daily, long brisk walks into town, gardened, practiced yoga and meditation, and made her own nut butters and used a vibrating machine on her feet to "increase circulation."

With an eternal smile on her face, she approached each day with a light heart, moved easefully and joyfully throughout her day. Her laughter was contagious and when I asked her "secret" to her vitality, good mood and excellent health, she replied, "Keep moving!" Cleo embodied the spirit of eternal youth. I often reflect on all she taught me and from time to time use her breakfast blend recipe of sprouts, greens, fruit, Rejuvelac (a cultured probiotic-rich drink), aloe, green algae powder, flax seed powder smoothie.

Movement vs exercise

Let's face it, a lot of us don't enjoy exercise. The idea of a gym surrounded by sweaty men or pedaling until we drop in a SoulCycle class can be a source of dread rather than inspiration.

But movement, be it dance, Zumba, belly dancing or tai chi, unleashes endorphins and leaves one feeling inspired, vibrant and joyful. My advice? Ignore the workouts that bore you and embrace movement.

All types of activity, aerobic or anaerobic contribute to improved mood and stress reduction. Endorphins, the body's feel-good neurotransmitters, are released during movement creating a natural high and sense of well-being. Movement, such as tai chi, is also a form of meditation in motion. Often, it's the combination of music we play, the company of other dancers that also uplifts our spirit.

When one engages in movement the mind is focused, leaving little time for thoughts of life's stressful events.

Movement has been proven to decrease levels of depression, anxiety and improve self-esteem. Yoga, or stretching movements, have also been proven to decrease tension and anxiety.

Why move vs sitting all day?

There are significant benefits to moving from increased circulation to lymphatic flow (the body's detoxification pathways), bone density, heart health, immune function, better digestion, improved sleep and reduced stress levels just to name a few. Exercise can be as effective as medication and psychotherapies. Regular exercise may boost mood by increasing a brain protein called BDNF that helps nerve fibers grow.

Harvard Medical School professor Srini Pillay, M.D. writes in a 2016 Harvard Health blog that "frequent yoga practice can reduce the severity of symptoms in post-traumatic stress disorder to the point that some people no longer meet the criteria for this diagnosis. Changing your posture, breathing, and rhythm can all change your brain, thereby reducing stress, depression, and anxiety, and leading to a feeling of well-being."

Studies also have shown that moving in synchrony with someone else, also improves your self-esteem. It's even been demonstrated that synchronizing your movement with others makes you like them more. You also cooperate more with them and feel more charitable towards them.

This may be why dance movement therapy can help depressed patients feel better.

What types of movement do we need?

Cardio exercise involves increasing your heart rate to burn energy and fat. Anything that achieves that result is considered cardio. It doesn't have to be a five-mile run or a ten-mile bike ride. A set of earphones and some hot dance music in your bedroom can turn a gloomy morning into a bath of bright light.

Movement can be as simple as a brisk daily walk for 30-45 minutes moving your arms freely while absorbing light from nature just as plants do. Rain or shine walking can also be a time to reflect, set intentions, receive guidance or repeat a mantra. Cleo held a strand of beads in her hand as she walked to and from town reminding herself of the divine nature within and without. Tulsi beads or rose quartz beads can be used for this practice. In Sanskrit, this is known as *japa*, — Christians also have the similar practice of rosary.

After walking, consider trying 25 low impact jumping jacks, ten knees bent pushups and twenty crossover knee to chest, elbow to knee movements, which help to balance the right and left brain.

Some immediate benefits of movement internally and externally are improved immune function, better digestion, and disease prevention. The aging process can be slowed down by freedom of movement. B. K. S. Iyengar was the perfect example of this. He created a style and approach to yoga that has become known as "Iyengar Yoga" and likely has done more than anyone to bring yoga to the West. Iyengar lived until 94 years old and practiced and taught yoga daily at his yoga institute in Pune India.

Movement can have a beneficial effect on immune function. Frequent tai chi has been shown to increase T-lymphocyte count in the body. Moderate intensity exercise has revealed beneficial effects on leukocyte or white blood cell concentration in the blood following exercise.

What is hatha yoga?

Hatha yoga is a series of movements creating internal and external strength, improved cardiovascular function, and an awareness of movement by synchronizing the postures with the breath. The ultimate purpose of yoga is to prepare the body to sit for meditation. Many attribute the origin of yoga as first articulated in Patanjali's Yoga Sutras, widely regarded as the authoritative text on yoga. Its collection of aphorisms, outline the eight limbs of yoga. These "threads" of wisdom offer guidelines for living a meaningful and purposeful life while the yoga we know today as "hatha yoga," represents only one of yoga's eight limbs.

Restorative yoga is for those who "do" too much and "rest too little." Yes, that may sound like all of us. It is the antithesis of hot yoga, vinyasa or any yoga that is more athletic in nature. You can linger in a restorative pose for 10 or 15 minutes, giving your body and mind plenty of time to relax and replenish.

In truth, restorative yoga is just that—restorative. Even if you have a regular, vigorous style yoga practice, teachers like Iyengar also recommend including a restorative session at the end of each week.

What is tai chi?

Tai chi is a gentle form of exercise that can help maintain strength, flexibility, and balance, and could be the perfect movement enhancing activity for the rest of your life. Tai chi is often described as "meditation in motion." I often wonder what our school system would be like if children practiced tai chi for fifteen minutes before the bell rang.

Tai chi, also transliterated in English as *taiji*, is an ancient Chinese martial art of slow, deliberate movements that have been shown to enhance physical and emotional health. It's a perfect practice at any age. It's common to see people in parks in China at dawn who are well into their 70s, moving with the fluidity of youthful dancers.

Some of the medical and emotional benefits of tai chi include:

- Improved mood, and lower levels of depression, hypertension, stress, and anxiety.
- Increased energy and stamina.
- Enhanced balance, flexibility, and agility.
- Lower blood pressure and improved heart health.

In *Brain, Behavior, and Immunity*, UCLA's Dr. Michael R. Irwin, director of the Cousins Center for Psychoneuroimmunology and Semel Institute for Neuroscience, and his colleague, Dr. Julienne E. Bower, reviewed 26 randomized controlled trials on the efficacy of tai chi, qigong, and meditation to reduce inflammation.

Their finding? Even after relatively short (6 weeks) interventions, study participants reversed cellular and genomic markers of inflammation. That's fantastic news since inflammation is associated with symptoms such as fatigue, insomnia, depression, and pain.

Of course, tai chi, qigong, yoga, and meditation—practices that include specific movements or postures, coordinated breathing, and mental focus—also require no drugs, and have no side effects—except, of course, an increased sense of calm and well-being.

These results are based on studies where participants learned only very basic and shortened set of tai chi moves so imagine the greater benefits of practicing an entire tai chi form. For true masters, tai chi is an internal exercise that does not rely on physical strength but relies on activating the chi, the flowing life energy that in Chinese philosophy is thought to be inherent in all things.

Tai chi is widely taught in the U.S. and it is worthwhile to find a qualified instructor. You may wish to visit more than one class to discover the group most suitable for you.

Speaking of moving like water, swimming, with its nominal resistance on the joints, brings together a host of benefits: cardio, flexibility, and fun. Salt pools vs chlorine pools are now more of the norm, leaving you less prone to the effects of chlorine or other chemicals.

What can I do if I work from home?

Of course, tai chi, yoga, and meditation can all be practiced at home. In addition, I'm a fan of something called a "rebounder," which can provide numerous health benefits in just five to ten minutes a day. Like a trampoline, a rebounder is tightly wound – it's only a small move upward from the apparatus – and its gentle bounce makes it easy on the joints. Some of its benefits include:

Boosts lymphatic drainage and immune function.

- Great for skeletal system and increasing bone mass.
- Helps improve digestion.

It's been shown to be twice as effective as running without the extra stress on the ankles and knees.

There are many choices of rebounders and prices range from $45 to $400. I recommend checking the ratings and finding a good quality rebounder.

Dance

Dance as if no one is looking, sing as if no one is listening.

Be it ballroom dance, salsa, African, Zumba, jazz, belly dance, ballet, hip hop or Sufi dancing, the benefits of dance on our bodies and brains, as mentioned earlier, are simply extraordinary.

Gabrielle Roth's, 5Rythms dance is a dynamic movement process of being in your body that ignites creativity, community, and connection. When I first began studying healing, 5Rythms was beginning to take off and I was a happy participant during those early years. I found it released any emotions or negativity I was feeling and left me feeling inspired, joyful and ecstatic. You can now find 5Rythms dances across the U.S. and around the world. It certainly embodies the idea that "movement is the medicine." It can also foster a deep sense of community, playfulness, and self-expression.

Local groups may have different names, "Sweat Your Prayers" or "Fumbling Towards Ecstasy" but can be found by Googling, "5Rhythms."

Belly Dancing

Every woman should take a belly dancing class. I was amazed the first time I tried it. It was inspiring to see how comfortable and expressive women were, regardless of body size. My shyness quickly fell away from exposing my not so perfect midriff after two childbirths. I loved the bells, costumes, colors, glitter and beaded pink slippers.

Besides toning the belly (a nice benefit), belly dancing awakens the first and second chakra, increasing sexuality and passion. Anyone who needs a spark in this area—married, single, menopausal or postmenopausal—I highly recommend it. Most Western exercises tighten the hips while belly dancing loosens them. The dance is also a beautiful way to celebrate your feminine body as it is.

What about Pilates?

A friend said this about Pilates "I've been doing Pilates three times a week now for several months and it's been a true godsend for my health. It's been phenomenal in helping me with my alignment and awakening my whole kinetic chain from toes, ankles, knees, groin to shoulders, neck, and head."

Joseph Pilates, the inventor of the Pilates Method, studied many forms of movement from all walks of life. After years of dedication and research to find a workout that could restore people to neutral posture and alignment he created the Pilates Method. This series of movements when done properly can increase flexibility, balance, muscle control, and core strength. A skilled instructor can guide you every step of the way.

There is a vitality, a life force, an energy, a quickening that is translated through you into action, and because there is only one of you in all time, this expression is unique. And if you block it, it will never exist through any other medium and will be lost.
— Martha Graham

Life is the dancer and you are the dance.
— Eckhart Tolle, A New Earth: Awakening to Your Life's Purpose

Conclusion

egin where you begin. Yes, there's a lot of information and suggestions packed into this book. You don't have to follow all of it. What did you read that got you thinking, "That would help me!"

Then begin with that. Whether that is grabbing your paints, heading out more often for walks in nature or taking up a tai chi or meditation practice.

Listen to that quiet inner voice.

Unlike some Western medicines, the only risk from these approaches is excessive smiling. The key though is to take a first step. If you *only* read this book, helpful as the information is, without taking any action, it's not going to help.

But if you're like me, I find that even a small step can spark profound change. Maybe this week, you simply begin applying some high-quality essential oils and notice that it helps your mood. Who knows then what step you'll feel inspired to take the following week.

I'd love to hear from you and learn what's been helpful. I promise to post helpful links and new tools, techniques and resources on my website and weekly blog @ www. gedaliahhealingarts.com. Who knows, perhaps if you're in the Greater Atlanta area, we'll have the opportunity to work together in person or at one of my retreats.

I thank you and honor you for joining me on this journey. I definitely am still taking daily steps towards my own health and vibrancy. It means a lot to have other women like yourself on the path with me. I send you my blessings and love on your pilgrimage.

Further Reading

Ayurveda- some of my favorites

The Science of Self-Healing, Vasant Lad
The Complete Book of Ayurvedic Home Remedies, Vasant Lad
The Ayurvedic Cookbook, Amadea Morningstar
The Three Season Diet, John Douillard
What Are You Hungry For? Dr. Deepak Chopra
Absolute Beauty, Pratima Raichur

Chakras- detailed books

Chakras and Their Archetypes, Ambika Wauters
Wheels of Light, Rosalyn Bruyere
Creating Mandalas for Insight, Healing and Self Expression, S.F. Fincher
Chakras- Energy Centers of Transformation, H.Johari
Mandalas- Luminous Symbols for Healing, Judith Cornell
Anatomy of the Spirit, Caroline Myss
You Can Heal your Life, Louise Hay
The Mystic Spiral, Journey of the Soul, Jill Purce
Healing with Music and Color- A Beginner's Guide, by Mary Bassano

Women's Wisdom (gems)

A Woman's Worth, Marianne Williamson
A Return to Love, Marianne Williamson
Living With Joy, Sanaya Roman
All Women Are Healers, Diane Stein
God Wears Lipstick, Karen Berg

Creativity (a go-to for connecting with creativity and healing the inner child)- A true transformative process book.)

The Artist's Way, Julia Cameron

Mental/Emotional Well Being

Mind of Your Own, Dr. Kelly Brogan
Emotional Intelligence, Travis Bradberry, and Jean Greaves
The Empath's Survival Guide, Judith Orloff, M.D.
Brain's Way of Healing, Norman Doidge
Women's Bodies Women's Wisdom, Christiane Northrup, M.D.
It Didn't Start with You, Mark Wolynn
The 21 Day Belly Fix, Tasneem Bhatia, M.D.

Chinese Medicine

Healing with Whole Foods, Paul Pitchford

A few goodies to have:

Consciousness and Healing, Marilyn Schlitz
The Edgar Cayce Remedies, William A. McGarry, M.D.
The Healing Voice, Joy Gardner Gordon
A Woman's Book of Life. Joan Borysenko, Ph.D
Essential Oils Desk Reference, Dr. Gary Young
Light of Yoga, B.K.S Iyengar
Shakti Woman, Vicki Noble
Super Woman RX, Dr. Tasneem Bhatia

Meditation
Meditate, Swami Muktananda
Inner Treasures, Gurumayi Chidvilasananda

Recommended websites
Banyan Botanicals- https://www.banyanbotanicals.com/
The Ayurvedic Institute- http://www.ayurveda.com/
Siddha Yoga- http://www.siddhayoga.org
Centre Spring MD-http://www.centrespringmd.com
Gedaliah Healing Arts- http://www.gedaliahhealingarts.com
Mighty Words- Gali Kronenberg editor bygali@me.com
Gaia Television- Continue your evolution to consciousness with Gaia

Essential Oil Resources
Nature's Gifts- https://www.naturesgift.com/
Mountain Rose- https://www.mountainroseherbs.com
Young Living- https://www.youngliving.com/blog/

Join my weekly blog "Get Your Groove Back" @ http://gedaliah-healingarts.com
Pause by Gedalia Essential Oil Roll On- www.gedaliahhealingarts.com
Visit my art @gedaliahhealingarts.com

Lack of Sleep =
    Overeating
- Reduce chronic stress
- Daily Routine
-   Restores Natural
      Balance
- Mental Loop - we dont
  pay attention -
    unconscious
   " I am fine as I am
right now "
    the thought pattern
is not true
"I am the Source of my
  own inner healing "

Made in the USA
Columbia, SC
19 February 2018